How to Lose Belly Fat

Effective Belly Fat Loss Tips (Science Based)

Chris Flick

Table of Contents

Chapter One

Understanding Belly Fat

Belly fat, scientifically known as abdominal or visceral fat, is a type of fat that accumulates around the abdominal cavity. Subcutaneous fat and visceral fat are the two basic categories into which it can be divided.

1.1 Subcutaneous Fat:

The layer of fat directly beneath the skin is called subcutaneous fat. While excess subcutaneous fat can contribute to a flabby appearance, it is less concerning from a health perspective compared to visceral fat.

Subcutaneous fat can be found throughout the body, including the arms, thighs, and buttocks.

1.2 Visceral Fat:

Visceral fat, on the other hand, is stored deep within the abdominal cavity, surrounding internal organs such as the liver, pancreas, and intestines. Higher levels of visceral fat are associated with an increased risk of various health issues, including cardiovascular diseases, diabetes, and metabolic syndrome.

1.3 The Dangers of Excess Belly Fat:

Excess abdominal fat carries serious health hazards in addition to being an aesthetic issue. Visceral fat is metabolically active, releasing inflammatory substances and hormones that can disrupt the normal functioning of organs. This can lead to insulin resistance, elevated blood sugar levels, and an increased risk of chronic diseases.

1.4 Body Mass Index (BMI) and Waist-to-Hip Ratio:

Body Mass Index (BMI) is a widely used tool to estimate body fat based on weight and height. While it provides a general indication of whether a person is underweight, normal weight, overweight, or obese, it does not differentiate between fat and muscle mass.

The waist-to-hip ratio is a more specific measurement that considers the distribution of fat in the body. A higher ratio indicates a greater concentration of fat around the abdomen and is associated with an increased risk of cardiovascular diseases.

The Science Behind Fat Loss

Understanding the science behind fat loss is essential for developing an effective strategy to shed excess belly fat and improve overall health. Fat loss involves a combination of physiological processes, including metabolism, hormonal regulation, and energy balance.

2.1 Metabolism and Energy Balance:

Metabolism is the set of chemical processes that occur within the body to maintain life. When it comes to fat loss, metabolism plays a central role. It involves two main components:

2.1.1 Basal Metabolic Rate (BMR):

BMR represents the energy expended at rest to maintain basic physiological functions such as breathing, circulation, and cell production. The higher your BMR, the more calories your body burns at rest, contributing to fat loss.

2.1.2 Energy Balance:

Fat loss occurs when the number of calories expended exceeds the number of calories consumed. Creating a calorie deficit, either through increased physical activity or reduced calorie intake, prompts the body to utilize stored fat for energy.

2.2 Hormones and Fat Storage:

Hormones are essential for controlling how fat is stored and used. The pancreas secretes insulin, which helps cells take up glucose. Elevated insulin levels, often associated with high-carbohydrate diets, can promote fat storage.

2.2.1 Insulin Resistance:

Over time, constant exposure to high insulin levels can lead to insulin resistance, where cells become less responsive to insulin's effects. This condition is linked to increased fat storage, particularly in the abdominal area.

2.2.2 Leptin and Ghrelin:

The hormones leptin and ghrelin control hunger and fullness. Leptin signals the brain when you're full, while ghrelin stimulates hunger. Imbalances in these hormones can contribute to overeating and weight gain.

2.3 Macronutrients and Fat Loss:

The composition of your diet plays a crucial role in fat loss. Understanding the role of macronutrients; carbohydrates, proteins, and fats is key to creating a well-balanced and effective nutrition plan.

2.3.1 Carbohydrates:

Carbohydrates provide a primary source of energy. Choosing complex carbohydrates with a low glycemic index can help stabilize blood sugar levels and prevent excessive insulin spikes.

2.3.2 Proteins:

Proteins are essential for muscle maintenance and repair. A protein-rich diet can help preserve lean muscle mass during weight loss and contribute to a feeling of fullness.

2.3.3 Fats:

Healthy fats, such as those found in avocados, nuts, and olive oil, play a crucial role in hormone production and satiety. Including these fats in your diet can support overall health and aid in fat loss.

2.4 Exercise for Fat Loss:

Physical activity is a cornerstone of any effective fat loss plan. Exercise contributes to calorie expenditure, improves metabolic rate, and enhances overall well-being.

2.4.1 Cardiovascular Exercise:

Aerobic exercises like running, cycling, and swimming can help burn calories and promote fat loss. High-intensity interval training (HIIT) is particularly effective in this regard.

2.4.2 Strength Training:

Building lean muscle mass through strength training not only contributes to a higher BMR but also enhances the overall aesthetic appearance of the body.

Chapter Two

Nutrition for Belly Fat Loss

3.1 The importance of a balanced diet

A balanced diet is a cornerstone of overall health and well-being, playing a crucial role in supporting various bodily functions, maintaining energy levels, and promoting sustainable weight management. In the context of losing belly fat, a balanced diet provides the essential nutrients needed to optimize metabolism and support fat loss.

1. Nutrient Variety for Optimal Health:

A balanced diet ensures that the body receives a wide range of essential nutrients, including:

- Macronutrients:

  - Carbohydrates: Provide energy for daily activities and support proper brain function.

  - Proteins: Essential for building and repairing tissues, including lean muscle mass.

  - Fats: Necessary for hormone production, cell structure, and absorption of fat-soluble vitamins.

- Micronutrients:

   - Vitamins: Play vital roles in metabolism, immune function, and various physiological processes.

   - Minerals: Essential for bone health, nerve function, and the regulation of fluid balance.

2. Energy Balance and Caloric Control:

A balanced diet helps maintain an appropriate caloric intake to support energy needs while preventing excess calorie consumption:

- Portion Control: Including a variety of foods in appropriate portions helps regulate calorie intake, preventing overeating and supporting weight management.

- Nutrient Density: Choosing nutrient-dense foods ensures that the body receives essential nutrients without excess calories, promoting satiety and overall health.

3. Blood Sugar Regulation:

Balancing carbohydrates, proteins, and fats in a meal contributes to stable blood sugar levels, which is crucial for preventing insulin spikes and reducing the risk of fat storage:

- Complex Carbohydrates: Choosing whole grains, fruits, and

vegetables provides a steady release of glucose, supporting sustained energy levels.

- Protein: Including protein in meals helps slow down the absorption of carbohydrates, preventing rapid spikes in blood sugar.

- Healthy Fats: Incorporating healthy fats helps regulate appetite and supports blood sugar control.

4. Support for Metabolism and Fat Loss:

A balanced diet supports metabolic processes, providing the nutrients needed for efficient energy utilization and fat metabolism:

- Lean protein: Foods rich in protein contribute to the preservation of lean muscle mass and support a higher basal metabolic rate (BMR).

- Healthy fats: Including sources of omega-3 fatty acids and monounsaturated fats can help with hormone production and promote fat loss.

5. Mental and emotional well-being:

A balanced diet not only benefits physical health, but also plays a role in mental and emotional well-being:

- Mood regulation: Nutrient-rich foods contribute to the production of neurotransmitters that regulate mood and reduce the risk of emotional overeating.

- Sustainability: A balanced diet that includes a variety of foods is more likely to be sustainable in the long term and promote a positive relationship with food.

6. Disease prevention and long-term health:

A well-balanced diet is associated with a lower risk of chronic diseases, including cardiovascular disease, diabetes and some cancers:

- Antioxidants: Fruits and vegetables, rich in antioxidants, help protect cells from damage and reduce inflammation.

- Fiber: Whole grains, fruits, and vegetables provide fiber that supports digestive health and may contribute to weight management.

3.2 Macronutrients and their role in fat metabolism

Carbs, proteins, and fats are examples of macronutrients, and they are all necessary for a diet that is balanced. Understanding the specific roles of each macronutrient in fat metabolism is key to designing an effective nutritional plan to support weight loss, especially in reducing belly fat.

1.1 Carbohydrates:

- Primary source of energy: Carbohydrates are the primary source of energy for the body. When consumed, they are broken down into glucose, which is used as fuel.

- Blood sugar regulation: Complex carbohydrates, such as whole grains and vegetables, ensure a steady release of glucose and prevent a rapid rise in blood sugar. This in turn helps regulate insulin secretion and reduces the risk of excessive fat storage.

- Exercise Fuel: Carbohydrates are essential for high-intensity exercise and can support effective exercise and contribute to overall calorie expenditure.

1.2 Proteins:

- Preservation of muscle mass: Adequate protein intake is decisive for the preservation of pure muscle mass, especially when losing weight. Muscle tissue contributes to a higher basal metabolic rate (BMR) and supports fat metabolism.

- Thermic effect: Protein has a higher thermic effect of food compared to carbohydrates and fats. This means that the body uses more energy to digest and process protein, which further contributes to overall calorie expenditure.

- Satiety: Protein-rich foods promote a feeling of fullness and satiety, reduce the likelihood of overeating and support weight management.

1.3 Fats:

- Hormone production: Dietary fats, especially healthy fats such as omega-3 fatty acids, play a key role in hormone production. Hormones such as leptin and insulin influence appetite regulation and fat storage.

- Energy source: Fats serve as a secondary source of energy, especially during lower intensity activities or periods of low carbohydrate availability. The body can draw energy from stored fat.

- Cell structure: Fats are an integral part of cell membranes and play a role in the structure and function of cells throughout the body.

1.4 Optimization of macronutrient ratios:

- Balancing ratios: Achieving a balanced ratio of carbohydrates, proteins and fats in food promotes overall health and helps maintain caloric balance leading to fat metabolism.

- Individual variability: The ideal ratio of macronutrients may vary among individuals based on factors such as age, gender, activity level, and metabolic rate. Personalization of macronutrient intake can optimize fat metabolism.

1.5 Timing and composition of food:

- Pre-workout nutrition: Consuming a combination of carbohydrates and protein before exercise provides the energy needed for exercise and supports the preservation of muscle mass.

- Post-workout nutrition: Including protein and carbohydrates in post-workout meals helps with muscle recovery, replenishes glycogen stores and supports fat metabolism during the recovery phase.

3.3 Foods that promote fat loss and should be avoided

Choosing the right foods is a critical aspect of any effective weight loss strategy. By incorporating nutrient-dense foods that boost your metabolism and avoiding those that contribute to excess calorie intake and fat storage, you can optimize your belly fat loss efforts.

1.1 Foods that promote weight loss:

- 1. Lean proteins:

- Sources: Lean beef, tofu, fish, poultry, turkey, and beans.

- Role: Supports the preservation of muscle mass, contributes to a higher basal metabolic rate (BMR) and promotes a feeling of fullness.

- 2. Whole grains:

- Sources: Quinoa, brown rice, oats, whole wheat.

- Role: Provides complex carbohydrates for sustained energy, stabilizes blood sugar and supports digestive health.

- 3. Fruits and vegetables:

- Sources: Berries, leafy greens, apples, broccoli, peppers.

- Role: Rich in fiber, vitamins and antioxidants, promotes satiety, supports metabolism and reduces inflammation.

- 4. Healthy fats:

  - Sources: Avocado, nuts, seeds, olive oil, fatty fish (salmon, mackerel).

  - Role: Supports the production of hormones, provides essential fatty acids and contributes to the feeling of fullness.

- 5. Low-fat dairy products or dairy alternatives:

  - Sources: Greek yogurt, low-fat milk, almond milk.

  - Role: High in protein and calcium, supporting muscle preservation and bone health.

- 6. Water:

  - Role: Staying hydrated promotes overall health, aids digestion and can help control appetite by preventing hunger caused by dehydration.

- 7. Green tea:

  - Role: Contains antioxidants and catechins that can improve metabolism and promote fat breakdown.

1.2 Foods to avoid or limit:

- 1. Refined carbohydrates:

  - Examples: white bread, sweet cereals, pastries.

  - Reason: Rapid rise in blood sugar, leading to insulin spikes and increased fat storage.

– 2. Sweetened drinks:

  - Examples: Soda, energy drinks, sugary drinks.

  - Reason: The high content of empty calories contributes to excessive sugar intake and does not ensure a feeling of satiety.

- 3. Processed and fried foods:

- Examples: Fast food, fried snacks, processed meat.

- Reason: Often high in unhealthy fats, sodium and additives, which contribute to inflammation and excess calorie intake.

- 4. High-calorie snacks:

  - Examples: Potato chips, candy bars, sweet snacks.

  - Reason: They tend to be high in calories and can lead to overconsumption.

- 5. Excessive alcohol:

  - Rationale: While moderate alcohol consumption may be

acceptable, excessive intake can contribute to increased calorie consumption and impaired judgment, leading to poor food choices.

- 6. Sugar and processed spices:

  - Examples: ketchup, sweet sauces, salad dressings.

  - Reason: It can add unnecessary calories, sugar and unhealthy fats to meals.

1.3 Strategies for smart food choices:

- 1. Portion control:

- Tip: Pay attention to portion sizes to avoid overeating, even with healthy foods.

- 2. Balanced meals:

- Tip: Include a combination of lean protein, whole grains, and vegetables in each meal for a balanced nutritional profile.

- 3. Meal timing:

- Tip: Consider timing nutrients around training to optimize energy levels and promote recovery.

- 4. Mindful eating:

- Tip: Pay attention to hunger and satiety signals and avoid distractions while eating.

3.4 The importance of portion control

Portion control is a fundamental aspect of a successful and sustainable approach to weight management and weight loss. Understanding the importance of portion control can help you make informed decisions about the amount of food you consume, supporting your goals of reducing belly fat and improving overall health.

1.1 Prevention of overeating:

- Caloric Intake: Portion size control helps manage total caloric intake and prevents the consumption of excess calories that can contribute to weight gain and fat storage.

- Energy Balance: Achieving a balance between the calories you take in and the calories your body expends is critical to weight maintenance and fat loss.

- Mindful Eating: Portion control promotes mindful eating, allowing you to savor and enjoy your food while being aware of your body's hunger and fullness.

1.2 Weight loss support:

- Caloric deficit: To lose weight, you need to create a caloric deficit, which means you consume fewer calories than your body puts out. Portion control helps you regulate your calorie intake and makes it easier to create a calorie deficit for effective fat loss.

- Sustainability: Portion control is a sustainable and realistic approach to weight management, making it more likely that individuals will stick to their diet plans long-term.

1.3 Explanation of portion sizes:

- Portion standardization: Understanding standard portion sizes will allow you to make a more accurate assessment of your calorie intake and ensure that you are not underestimating the caloric content of your meals.

- Nutrient intake: Proper portion control ensures a balance of macronutrients and micronutrients promotes overall health and promotes optimal nutrient intake.

1.4 Portion Control Tools:

- Measuring cups and scales: Using measuring cups can help you become familiar with appropriate portion sizes, especially when cooking at home.

- Visual cues: Learning to visually estimate portion sizes, such as recognizing a serving of protein or a cup of vegetables, can be a valuable skill when dining or when measuring tools are not available.

- Plate composition: Divide your plate into sections and allocate space for protein, carbohydrates and vegetables. This visual aid can guide portion control.

1.5 Practical tips for portion control:

- Eat mindfully: Pay attention to your dining experience and focus on the flavors and textures of your food. Avoid distractions such as television or electronic devices.

- Use smaller plates: Choosing smaller plates can create the illusion of a fuller plate, helping you feel satisfied with smaller portions.

- Slow down: Eating slowly allows your body to register feelings of fullness, making you less likely to overeat.

- Listen to hunger and fullness signals: Pay attention to your body's hunger and fullness signals and stop eating when you feel full.

Chapter Three

Effective Exercise Strategies
The role of cardio in burning calories

Cardiovascular exercise, commonly known as cardio, is a key component of any comprehensive weight loss plan. Understanding the role of cardio in burning calories and promoting overall health is essential to designing an effective exercise routine that supports your goals to lose belly fat.

4.1 Caloric expenditure and weight loss:

- Caloric deficit: Weight loss occurs when the number of calories consumed exceeds the number of calories burned. Cardiovascular exercise contributes to caloric expenditure, helping to create the caloric deficit necessary for fat loss.

- Increased energy consumption: Engaging in cardio increases the body's energy demands, which leads to the use of stored fat as a fuel source. This process supports the breakdown of fat stores and contributes to weight loss.

4.2 Types of cardiovascular exercise:

- 1. Low Intensity Steady State (LISS):

  - Example: Walking, recreational cycling.

  - Role: Sustained moderate intensity activity that primarily depends on aerobic metabolism. LISS is accessible to individuals at various fitness levels.

- 2. High Intensity Interval Training (HIIT):

  - Example: Intervals of intense exercise (e.g. sprinting) followed by periods of rest or low-intensity activity.

  - Role: Alternating between high and low intensity maximizes calorie burn during exercise and can increase post-exercise metabolic rate.

- 3. Cardio lesson:

  - Example: Spinning, aerobics, dance cardio.

  - Role: Group classes provide a structured and motivating environment, combining cardio with strength and flexibility exercises.

- 4. Cardio machines:

  - Example: Treadmill, elliptical bike, stationary bike.

  - Role: The use of machines offers a controlled environment

that allows individuals to adjust intensity and monitor performance.

4.3 Cardio and Belly Fat:

- Reduction of visceral fat: Cardiovascular exercise has been associated with a reduction of visceral fat, the fat stored around the internal organs, which is especially important for reducing belly fat.

- Consistent calorie burn: Regular cardio sessions contribute to a consistent and sustained calorie burn and promote fat loss over time.

4.4 Effective Cardio Strategy:

- Frequency: Aim for at least 150 minutes of moderate-intensity cardio or 75 minutes of vigorous-intensity cardio per week, as recommended by health guidelines. Gradually increase the duration and intensity.

- Variety: Incorporate different cardio activities to engage different muscle groups and prevent monotony. This can include a combination of aerobic exercise, classes and outdoor activities.

- Progression: Challenge yourself by gradually increasing intensity, duration or incorporating interval training. This progression stimulates continuous adaptation and improves cardiovascular fitness.

- Consistency: Consistent and regular cardio sessions are key to achieving and maintaining weight loss. Establishing a routine that fits your lifestyle increases adherence.

4.5 Cardio and General Health:

- Cardiovascular health: As the name suggests, cardiovascular exercise benefits the heart and circulatory system and reduces the risk of cardiovascular disease.

- Mood and stress management: Cardio releases endorphins,

promotes positive mood and helps manage stress, which can be beneficial for overall well-being.

- Improved sleep: Regular cardio has been linked to improved sleep quality, which contributes to better overall health.

Strength training to build muscle and increase metabolism

Strength training, also known as resistance or strength training is a key part of a well-rounded weight loss plan. In addition to its muscle-building and toning benefits, strength training plays an important role in boosting metabolism and promoting overall health.

1. Building Muscle and Losing Fat:

- Lean muscle mass: Strength training helps build and maintain lean muscle mass. Unlike fat, muscle tissue is metabolically active and contributes to a higher basal metabolic rate (BMR). This means that even at rest, individuals with more muscle will burn more calories.

- Caloric expenditure: Intense strength training can increase post-exercise oxygen consumption (EPOC), leading to increased calorie burning in the hours following exercise. This contributes to the overall caloric deficit necessary for fat loss.

2. Increase in metabolism:

- Basal Metabolic Rate (BMR): Strength training increases BMR by promoting muscle growth. With more muscle mass, the body requires more energy at rest, which contributes to a higher metabolic rate.

- Afterburn Effect: Intense strength training creates an "afterburn" effect, where the body continues to burn calories in the period after exercise. This is due to the energy required for muscle recovery and regeneration.

- Insulin sensitivity: Strength training increases insulin sensitivity and improves the body's ability to regulate blood sugar. Improved insulin sensitivity may contribute to better fat metabolism and reduced fat storage.

3. Types of strength training:

- 1. Resistance exercises:

  - Examples: Weight lifting, exercises with your own weight (squats, lunges, push-ups).

  - Role: Targets specific muscle groups, promotes strength and hypertrophy.

- 2. Weighted high-intensity interval training (HIIT):

  - Example: Combination of short series of intense exercises with weights.

  - Role: Includes cardio and strength elements for an effective workout.

- 3. Circuit training:

  - Example: Alternating different strength exercises with minimal rest.

- Role: Improves cardiovascular fitness while building strength.

- 4. Functional training:

  - Example: Exercises that mimic real-life movements.

  - Role: Improves overall functional strength and helps prevent injuries.

4. Incorporating strength training into your routine:

- Frequency: Aim for at least two to three strength training sessions per week, allowing for sufficient recovery between sessions.

- Progressive Overload: Gradually increase the resistance, repetitions or intensity of your strength training to continuously challenge your muscles and promote growth.

- Full Body Workout: Incorporate exercises targeting different muscle groups into each workout to ensure a balanced and comprehensive approach.

- Rest and Recovery: Allow yourself enough time to rest and recover to prevent overtraining and optimize muscle recovery.

5. Nutrition for strength training:

- Protein intake: Ensure adequate protein intake to support muscle recovery and growth. Protein-rich foods or supplements may be beneficial.

- Hydration: Stay hydrated to support overall performance and recovery during strength training.

- Balanced diet: Maintain a balanced diet with a mix of carbohydrates, protein and healthy fats to give you the energy you need to exercise and promote overall health.

6. Benefits Beyond Fat Loss:

- Bone health: Strength training helps improve bone density and reduces the risk of osteoporosis.

- Joint health: Properly performed strength training can improve joint stability and reduce the risk of injury.

- Mental health: Strength training is associated with improved mood, reduced stress and increased cognitive function.

High intensity interval training (HIIT) for effective fat burning

High-intensity interval training (HIIT) has gained popularity for its effectiveness in burning calories, promoting fat burning, and improving cardiovascular fitness. Understanding the principles and benefits of HIIT can help you incorporate this effective exercise approach into your weight loss plan.

1. What is HIIT?

- Interval structure: HIIT involves alternating between short intense bursts of exercise and periods of rest or lower intensity activity.

- Work-Rest Ratio: Common work-rest ratios include 30 seconds of intense exercise followed by 30 seconds of rest, or

1 minute of intense exercise
followed by 1 minute of rest.

- Adaptability: HIIT can be
adapted to a variety of exercises,
including running, cycling,
bodyweight exercises and
strength training.

2. Benefits of HIIT for fat
burning:

- 1. Increased caloric
expenditure:

  - Afterburn Effect: HIIT induces
excess post-exercise oxygen
consumption (EPOC), which leads
to continued calorie burning after
the workout.

- Efficiency: Shorter HIIT
sessions can burn more calories
compared to traditional steady-
state cardio.

- 2. Fat oxidation:

  - Improved metabolism: HIIT
has been shown to increase the
body's ability to oxidize fat for
energy during training and
recovery.

- 3. Preservation of lean muscle
mass:

  - Resistance to muscle loss:
HIIT has been shown to be
effective in preserving lean
muscle mass, which is essential

for maintaining a higher basal metabolic rate (BMR).

- 4. Time efficiency:

  - Short workouts: HIIT workouts are often shorter than traditional cardio workouts, making them a time-efficient option for individuals with busy schedules.

3. Types of HIIT training:

- 1. Cardio HIIT:

  - Example: Sprinting or cycling with maximum effort in short intervals.

  - Role: Increases heart rate and supports cardiovascular fitness.

- 2. Bodyweight HIIT:

- Example: Burpees, jumping jacks, mountain climbers.

  - Role: Targets multiple muscle groups, promotes strength and endurance.

- 3. Strength-based HIIT:

  - Example: Combination of strength exercises with short rest intervals.

  - Role: Builds strength and cardiovascular fitness at the same time.

- 4. Tabata:

  - Structure: For four minutes, alternate between 20 seconds of vigorous exercise and 10 seconds of rest.

  - Role: Short and intense, ideal for effective fat burning.

4. Incorporating HIIT into your routine:

- Frequency: Start with 2-3 HIIT sessions per week and gradually increase the intensity and duration.

- Progression: As fitness improves, increase intensity, duration or incorporate more challenging exercises.

- Warm-up and cool-down: Include a dynamic warm-up to prepare the body for intense exercise and a cool-down to facilitate recovery.

- Modifications: Adapt HIIT workouts to your fitness level and gradually increase the intensity as you get more fit.

5. Safety considerations:

- Consultation: If you have a pre-existing medical condition or concern, please consult a healthcare professional before starting HIIT.

- Form and technique: Ensure proper form during exercise to reduce the risk of injury. Start with a lower intensity and work your way up.

- Pay attention to your body. Be alert for symptoms of exhaustion or overdoing it. Adjust the intensity or rest if necessary.

6. Combining HIIT with other exercises:

- Complementary workouts: Combine HIIT with strength training and other forms of cardiovascular exercise for a well-rounded weight loss program.

- Variety: Incorporating different types of exercises prevents boredom and targets different muscle groups for balanced development.

Basic exercises focused on the abdominal muscles

Strengthening your core is a vital part of any comprehensive fitness routine, especially if the goal is to tone and define your abs. Focusing on a variety of core exercises helps improve stability, posture and overall functional strength. Here are effective core exercises targeting the abdominal muscles:

1. Basic core exercise:

- 1. Plank:

  - Position: Forearms and fingers on the ground, keep a straight line from head to heels.

- Focus: Engage the core, hold for 30 seconds to 1 minute.

- 2. Russian Twists:

  - Position: Sit with your knees bent, lean back slightly and rotate your torso while holding weights or clasped hands.

  - Focus: Engage the obliques; perform controlled twists for 15-20 reps on each side.

- 3. Bicycle cranks:

  - Position: Lie on your back, bring the opposite elbow and knee together in a cycling motion.

  - Focus: Engage the entire core; perform 15-20 reps on each side.

2. Advanced basic exercises:

- 4. Lifting legs in a sling:

  - Position: Hang on the pull-up bar and lift your legs straight up, avoid swinging.

  - Focus: Engage lower abs, perform 12-15 reps.

- 5. Plank variation (Side Plank, Spiderman Plank):

  - Side Plank: Support the body on one forearm and the side of one leg and keep the body straight.

  - Spiderman Plank: From a plank position, pull one knee to the elbow on the same side.

- Focus: The side plank focuses on the slopes; the Spiderman plank takes up the entire core.

- 6. Reverse Crunch:

  - Position: Lie on your back, pull your knees to your chest and lift your hips off the ground.

  - Focus: Engage lower abs, perform 15-20 reps.

3. Ball stability exercises:

- 7. Introducing the stability ball:

  - Position: Kneeling with hands on a stability ball, rolling the ball forward, stretching the body.

  - Focus: Engage core muscles, perform 12-15 reps.

- 8. Stability Ball Pike:

  - Position: Start in a plank position with your feet on a stability ball, lifting your hips toward the ceiling.

  - Focus: Engage lower abs, perform 12-15 reps.

4. Basic exercises based on Pilates:

- 9. Hundred:

  - Position: Lie on your back, lift your feet off the ground and pump your arms up and down.

  - Focus: Engage deep abdominal muscles, perform 100 pulses.

- 10. Pilates scissors:

- Position: Lie on your back, lift
one leg towards the ceiling while
the other hovers above the
ground.

- Focus: Engage the core and
switch legs in a scissor motion,
perform 15-20 reps.

5. Tips for effective basic
training:

- Consistency: For optimal
results, include core exercises 2-3
times a week in your routine.

- Correct form: Focus on quality
over quantity. Ensure proper form
to target the intended muscles
and avoid strain.

- Breathing: Maintain steady breathing during each exercise, exhale during the exertion phase.

- Progression: Gradually increase the difficulty of the exercises as your core strength improves.

Chapter Four

Lifestyle Changes for Sustainable Results

Sustainable fat loss goes beyond diet and exercise; it involves adopting healthy lifestyle habits that promote long-term well-being. Making these lifestyle changes can improve your overall quality of life while promoting lasting results on your belly fat loss journey.

1. Prioritizing sleep:

- Quality sleep: Aim for 7-9 hours of quality sleep each night. Lack of sleep can disrupt hormonal balance, affect hunger hormones and increase cravings for unhealthy foods.

- Consistent sleep schedule: Maintain a consistent sleep schedule by going to bed and getting up at the same time every day. This helps regulate your body's internal clock.

- Create a peaceful environment: Make your bedroom sleep-friendly by keeping it cool, dark and quiet. Reduce screen time before bed to enhance the quality of your sleep.

2. Coping with stress:

- Mindfulness and relaxation techniques: Practice mindfulness, meditation or deep breathing exercises to manage stress. Chronic stress can lead to an increase in cortisol levels, which contributes to the storage of belly fat.

- Regular physical activity: Engage in activities you enjoy, such as walking, yoga or spending time in nature. Physical activity helps reduce stress and promotes overall well-being.

- Time Management: Prioritize tasks and set realistic goals so you don't feel overwhelmed. Effective time management contributes to reducing stress levels.

3. Stay hydrated:

- Water consumption: Drink enough water during the day. Staying hydrated promotes overall health, aids digestion, and can help control appetite.

- Limit sugary drinks: Avoid excessive consumption of sugary drinks. Choose water, herbal teas or infused water with natural flavors.

4. Careful eating:

- Enjoy your food: Take the time to savor and enjoy each meal. Eating mindfully allows you to recognize hunger and fullness signals, which prevents overeating.

- Limit distractions: Avoid distractions such as television or electronic devices while eating. Focus on the sensory experience of your food.

- Portion control: Use smaller plates and utensils to control portions. Listen to your body's signals about hunger and fullness.

5. Building a support system:

- Accountability: Share your goals with friends, family or a fitness buddy. Motivation and accountability can be obtained from having a support network.

- Join classes or groups: Consider joining fitness classes or groups to connect with like-minded individuals. This fosters a sense of community and encouragement.

6. Smart snacks:

- Nutrient-Dense Snacks: Choose nutrient-dense snacks like fruit, vegetables or a handful of nuts. These foods improve general health and offer long-lasting energy.

- Plan ahead: Prepare healthy snacks in advance so you don't reach for less nutritious options when you're hungry.

7. Balance and Moderation:

- Moderate Treats: Treat yourself to occasional treats or indulgences in moderation. Complete deprivation can lead to cravings and potentially undermine long-term success.

- Balanced diet: Aim for a balanced and varied diet that contains a mix of macronutrients and micronutrients. This promotes overall health and well-being.

8. Consistent physical activity:

- Engage in fun activities: Engage in physical activities that you enjoy to make exercise a sustainable part of your routine. This can include dancing, hiking, or playing sports.

- Consistency over intensity: Prioritize consistent physical activity over occasional intense workouts. Regular movement contributes to overall energy expenditure.

9. Setting realistic goals:

- S.M.A.R.T. Goals: Set specific, measurable, achievable, relevant and time-bound goals. This framework increases clarity and increases the likelihood of success.

- Celebrate Milestones: Recognize and celebrate small and significant successes along the way. Positive reinforcement promotes motivation.

Creating a Personal Plan

When embarking on a journey to lose belly fat, creating a personalized plan that integrates diet strategies, exercise routines and lifestyle modifications is key to achieving sustainable and effective results. Tailoring your approach to your individual preferences, goals and lifestyle will ensure a plan you can stick to long term.

1. Assess your goals:

- Define clear goals: Clearly outline your weight loss goals. Whether it's a certain amount of weight to lose, inches around your waist or reaching a certain level of fitness, clear goals provide direction.

- Consider timelines: Set realistic timelines for your goals. Understand that sustainable fat loss is a gradual process and striving for steady progress over time is more effective than quick, short-term fixes.

2. Assess your current lifestyle:

- Dietary habits: Assess your current eating habits, including meal timing, food choices and portion sizes. Determine potential adjustments and opportunities for improvement.

- Physical activity: Assess your current exercise routine, if any. Consider the type, frequency and intensity of your training. Identify areas where you can introduce or improve physical activity.

- Sleep and stress: Think about your sleep patterns and stress levels. Identify opportunities to improve sleep quality and implement stress management techniques.

3. Designing Your Personal Plan:

- Nutrition strategies:

  - Caloric intake: Calculate your daily caloric needs based on your goals, taking into account factors such as age, gender, weight and activity level.

  - Macronutrient Balancing: Determine the appropriate ratio of carbohydrates, proteins and fats to match your preferences and support your weight loss goals.

  - Meal timing: Consider incorporating strategies such as intermittent fasting or mindful eating based on your lifestyle and preferences.

- Exercise routine:

  - Cardiovascular exercise: Choose cardio activities that you enjoy, aim for at least 150 minutes per week of moderate-intensity exercise or 75 minutes of vigorous-intensity exercise.

  - Strength Training: Integrate strength training 2-3 times per week with a focus on full body workouts that target major muscle groups.

  - HIIT classes: Include 1-2 high intensity interval training (HIIT) per week for effective fat burning.

- Lifestyle modifications:

  - Sleep hygiene: Implement sleep hygiene practices such as maintaining a consistent sleep schedule and creating a conducive sleep environment.

  - Stress management: Incorporate stress-reducing activities such as mindfulness, meditation or yoga into your routine.

  - Hydration: Ensure adequate water intake throughout the day to support overall health and metabolism.

- Monitoring and adjustments:

- Regular evaluation: Regularly reassess your progress towards your goals. Adjust your plan as needed based on your results and evolving preferences.

- Mindful adaptation: Be flexible and adapt your plan to changing circumstances. Life is dynamic and your weight loss plan should be adaptable to different situations.

4. Building Habits for Long-Term Success:

- Gradual implementation: Roll out changes gradually to better adapt. Trying to overhaul your entire lifestyle overnight can be overwhelming and less sustainable.

- The secret is consistency: Long-term success requires consistency. Focus on building habits that align with your goals and focus on progress rather than perfection.

- Celebrate achievements: Recognize and celebrate your achievements, whether they are small milestones or major victories. Positive reinforcement increases motivation.

5. Seek professional guidance:

- Expert Consultation: Consider consulting a nutritionist, fitness

trainer, or healthcare professional
for personalized advice based on
your unique needs and
circumstances.

- Regular Check-ins: Schedule
regular check-ins with
professionals to review your
progress, receive guidance, and
make necessary adjustments to
your plan.

Chapter Five

Supplements and Their Role

Supplements can be a supportive addition to your fat loss journey, providing essential nutrients, improving metabolism and addressing potential deficiencies. While no supplement can replace a balanced diet and regular exercise, some supplements can offer benefits in supporting your overall health and optimizing fat loss. It is essential to approach the use of supplements with caution and to consult a healthcare professional before introducing new products into your routine.

1. Common supplements for weight loss:

- 1. Protein supplements:

  - Role: Protein is crucial for muscle preservation and overall satiety. Protein supplements such as whey protein, casein, or plant-based supplements can help meet protein requirements, especially for those with increased physical activity.

- 2. Omega-3 fatty acids:

  - Role: Omega-3 fatty acids support overall health and may have anti-inflammatory effects. Fish oil supplements may be beneficial for individuals with low fish consumption.

- 3. Green tea extract:

  - Role: Green tea extract contains compounds such as catechins that can support metabolism and fat oxidation. It is often included in weight loss supplements.

- 4. Caffeine:

  - Role: Caffeine is a stimulant that can increase energy levels, increase alertness and potentially increase metabolism. It is commonly found in fat burning supplements and pre-workout formulas.

- 5. Fiber supplements:

  - Role: Adequate intake of fiber supports digestion promotes satiety and can help with weight management. Fiber supplements such as psyllium or glucomannan may be helpful for those trying to meet their fiber needs through food alone.

- 6. Vitamin D:

  - Role: Vitamin D plays a role in overall health and may influence weight management. Individuals with low sun exposure or inadequate dietary intake may benefit from supplementation.

- 7. BCAA (branched chain amino acids):

- Role: BCAAs, including leucine, isoleucine and valine, are essential amino acids that play a role in muscle protein synthesis. BCAA supplementation may promote muscle preservation during periods of calorie restriction.

2. Considerations before using supplements:

- Consult a healthcare professional: Consult a healthcare professional before incorporating any supplements, especially if you have an underlying medical condition or are taking medication.

- Individual needs: The need for supplements varies among individuals. Factors such as age, gender, dietary preferences and overall health should be taken into account.

- Product quality: Choose reputable brands and products that undergo third-party quality and purity testing. Ensuring the safety and effectiveness of supplements is essential.

- Dosage and Timing: Follow the recommended dosage and directions for each supplement.

Pay attention to timing, as some supplements are more effective when taken with food or at certain times of the day.

3. The role of a balanced diet:

- Primary source of nutrients: Although supplements can provide specific nutrients, they should not replace a balanced and varied diet. Whole foods offer a wider spectrum of nutrients, including fiber and phytonutrients.

- Nutritional synergy: Nutrients in whole foods often work synergistically to provide greater health benefits than isolated supplements. Focus on favoring nutrient-dense and whole-food sources.

- Hydration: Adequate hydration is essential for overall health and can promote fat loss. Water should be the primary beverage of choice.

4. Sustainable lifestyle habits:

- Focus on real foods: Emphasize a diet rich in nutrient-dense whole foods, including fruits, vegetables, lean protein, whole grains, and healthy fats.

- Regular physical activity: Exercise is an essential part of any weight loss plan.

Supplements should complement, not replace, a well-rounded fitness routine.

- Sleep and Stress Management: Prioritize quality sleep and stress management as an integral part of your fat loss journey.

5. Monitoring and Editing:

- Regular evaluation: Regularly reassess your progress and adjust your supplement regimen if needed. Track changes in body composition, energy levels and overall well-being.

- Professional Advice: Consult nutritionists, dietitians or fitness experts for personalized advice on supplement use based on your individual needs and goals.

Overcoming plateaus and challenges

Plateaus and challenges are common aspects of any fat loss journey. Understanding how to overcome these obstacles and implementing effective strategies can help you overcome obstacles and continue to achieve your goals. Here, we'll explore the various challenges you may encounter and offer strategies to overcome them.

1. Plateau identification:

- Weight loss has stalled: If your weight loss has stalled for several weeks despite constant efforts, you may have hit a plateau. Plateaus are often a normal part of the fat loss process.

- Decreased motivation: A decrease in motivation or adherence to your plan may indicate the need for adjustments. Identifying the root cause of reduced motivation is essential.

- Lack of progress in training: If you notice a lack of progress in training, such as no improvement in strength or endurance, this may be a sign of stagnation.

2. Common Challenges and Solutions:

- 1. Adjusting the diet:

  - Challenge: Eating too many calories, even from healthy foods.

  - Solution: Reevaluate portion sizes, monitor food intake and watch out for hidden calories. Consider adjusting your macronutrient balance if necessary.

- 2. Insufficient physical activity:

  - Challenge: Sticking to the same exercise routine without progression.

- Solution: Increase the
intensity, duration or frequency of
your workouts. Incorporate new
exercises or try different forms of
exercise to challenge your body.

- 3. Lack of consistency:

  - Challenge: Inconsistency in
following a weight loss plan.

  - Solution: Restore consistency
by setting specific and achievable
goals. Break larger goals into
smaller, manageable tasks to
gain momentum.

- 4. Metabolic adaptation:

  - Challenge: The body can adapt
to a caloric deficit by slowing
down the metabolism.

- Solution: Consider cycling your caloric intake by incorporating a slightly higher caloric period (recovery) or adjusting your total caloric intake.

- 5. Emotional eating:

  - Challenge: emotional variables that result in overindulging or making bad dietary decisions.

  - Solution: Develop strategies to manage stress and emotional triggers. Engage in mindful eating and seek support from friends, family or a professional if needed.

- 6. Insufficient sleep:

- Challenge: Insufficient sleep can affect hormonal balance and metabolism.

- Solution: Prioritize quality sleep by establishing a consistent sleep routine, creating a comfortable sleep environment, and addressing factors affecting sleep.

- 7. Overtraining:

- Challenge: Excessive exercise without adequate recovery can hinder progress.

- Solution: Take regular rest days, prioritize recovery strategies like stretching and foam rolling, and listen to your body for signs of fatigue.

- 8. Hormonal imbalance:

  - Challenge: Hormonal changes, especially in women, can affect fat loss.

  - Solution: Consult a health care professional to evaluate and address hormonal imbalances. Focus on overall health through nutrition, exercise and stress management.

3. Breaking Platforms:

- Calorie cycling: Establishing periods of higher and lower calorie intake can help prevent metabolic adaptation and break plateaus.

- Change your exercise routine: Add variety to your exercise routine by incorporating new exercises, adjusting the intensity or trying different types of exercise.

- Reassessing Goals: Evaluate and possibly revise your weight loss goals. Setting new, realistic goals can provide renewed motivation and focus.

- Track and Adjust: Track your progress regularly and be willing to adjust your plan based on what's working and what's not.

This may include tweaking your diet, exercise routine, or other aspects of your plan.

- Mindfulness practices: Incorporate mindfulness techniques such as meditation or deep breathing to manage stress and emotional overeating.

4. Stay motivated:

- Celebrate victories without the scale: Recognize achievements beyond the scale, such as better energy levels, better sleep, or increased fitness.

- Rethink your "why": Remind yourself of the reasons you started your fat loss journey.

Connecting with your deeper motivations can reignite your commitment.

- Visualize Success: Use visualization techniques to imagine achieving your goals. Visualizing success can increase motivation and focus.

- Accountability: Share your goals with a friend, family member or fitness buddy who can provide support, encouragement and accountability.

5. Seeking professional advice:

- Professional Consultation: If you are facing persistent problems or have specific health concerns, consider seeking professional advice, such as a nutritionist, fitness trainer, or health care provider.

- Regular Check-ins: Schedule regular check-ins with professionals to review your progress, receive guidance, and make necessary adjustments to your plan.

Remember, it's important to consult a healthcare professional before making significant changes to your diet or exercise, especially if you have pre-existing health conditions.